SURVIVING TRICHOMONIASIS

Beginners Comprehensive Approach To Combating & Managing Trichomoniasis Outbreak Effectively

Nuel Nenji

Table of Contents

Introduction

"Trich," short for "trichomoniasis," is a common STI caused by a tiny parasite called Trichomonas vaginalis. Both sexes are susceptible to this infection, however women are more likely to experience noticeable symptoms due to the focus of the infection on the vaginal and urinary tract.

Some essential facts about trichomoniasis are as follows:

1. The most common route of transmission for trichomoniasis is through oral, anal, or genital intercourse. The infected person need not show any symptoms to transmit

the disease to their sexual partner or partners.

2. Despite the prevalence of trichomoniasis, many afflicted individuals remain asymptomatic. On the other hand, when symptoms do show up, they could include:

• Itching, burning, or redness in the female reproductive organs; frothy, yellow-green vaginal discharge with a foul odor; difficulty or pain during sexual activity; and increased urine frequency.

• In men, symptoms include genital itching or irritation, post-urination or ejaculatory burning, and occasionally a little discharge.

3. Several diagnostic procedures exist for trichomoniasis, including culture tests, nucleic acid amplification tests (NAATs) that detect the parasite's genetic material, and microscopic inspection of a vaginal or urethral swab.

4. Complications: If untreated, trichomoniasis can increase the likelihood of contracting or transferring other sexually transmitted infections (STIs), and in pregnant women, it may be linked to premature delivery or low birth weight.

5. Antibiotics, such as metronidazole or tinidazole, can be prescribed to treat trichomoniasis. Both sexual partners must get treatment at the same time to avoid reinfection.

6. Safe sex practices, such as the right and regular use of condoms, are the most effective means of preventing trichomoniasis and other sexually transmitted infections. Restricting one's access to sexual partners and routinely screening for sexually transmitted infections are other vital preventative measures.

Timely identification and treatment can reduce the risk of complications and stop the spread of trichomoniasis and other sexually transmitted infections (STIs). You should also tell your sexual partners so that they can get tested and, if necessary, receive treatment.

CHAPTER ONE
Trichomonas Vaginalis Life Cycle

The trichomoniasis-causing parasite, Trichomonas vaginalis, has a straightforward and multistage life cycle. Trichomonas vaginalis has the following stages in its life cycle:

• The trophozoite is the infectious and active stage of the parasite's life cycle. Single-celled trophozoites have flagella (whip-like structures) to propel them forward. They flourish in the hot and humid conditions of the urinary and vaginal systems of both sexes. It is possible for an infected person to spread the trophozoites to their sexual partner.

• As soon as they enter a new host, trophozoites seek out the epithelial cells covering the mucous membranes of the vaginal and urinary systems, where they attach and begin colonizing. They are able to attach to and remain in these cells thanks to structures like an undulating membrane and an axostyle.

• Multiplication: Once connected, trophozoites can divide into two identical copies of themselves through a process called binary fission. As a result, the parasite population grows within the host.

• When Trichomonas vaginalis is present, it can interact with host cells, which can set off an inflammatory reaction. Women in particular are more likely to have symptoms including itching, burning, and discharge if infected.

• Some trophozoites can change into a cyst-like structure termed pseudocysts in response to unfavorable conditions including a lack of nutrients or exposure to harsh settings. Pseudocysts may withstand harsh conditions and may even be able to live temporarily apart from the host.

• Trichomonas vaginalis can live in two different environments: extracellularly (outside host cells) and intracellularly (inside host cells). Although it is often found in the extracellular space, it can infrequently enter host cells.

• Sexual contact, whether it be vaginal, anal, or oral, is the primary mode of transmission for Trichomonas vaginalis. During childbirth, an infected mother can pass the virus on to her kid.

• Antibiotics like metronidazole and tinidazole are efficient against the trophozoite type, making them a good choice for treating trichomoniasis. Pseudocysts, unlike true cysts, may be more difficult to cure due to their resistance.

The development of reliable diagnostic tools and efficient treatment techniques for trichomoniasis relies on a thorough understanding of the life cycle of Trichomonas vaginalis. Preventing problems and spreading the infection requires prompt diagnosis and treatment.

The Signs And The Scrutiny

Trichomoniasis, caused by the parasite Trichomonas vaginalis, can cause a wide variety of symptoms, or sometimes no symptoms at all.

When symptoms do occur, they may manifest differently in males and females. In addition, a number of laboratory tests are routinely used to identify trichomoniasis.

Trichomoniasis Manifestations:

In Females:

- Many infected women report a foamy, yellow-green vaginal discharge, which may be particularly pungent.

- Symptoms of vaginal irritation include itchiness, redness, and pain.

- Urinary Burning: a painful or uncomfortable sensation when trying to urinate.

- Pain or distress experienced during sexual activity.

In Men:

- Some sick males may bleed from the penis, which is called a urethral discharge.

• Feelings of itchiness or irritation in the penis.

• When you urinate or ejaculate, you feel a scorching feeling.

Trichomoniasis is a sexually transmitted disease that can be passed on unwittingly by many infected people who do not exhibit any symptoms (asymptomatic).

Trichomoniasis testing and diagnosis:

Most often, laboratory testing are used to identify trichomoniasis. Here are some typical approaches to diagnosis:

• Examining a sample of discharge or secretions from the genitourinary tract under the microscope. If an infection with Trichomonas vaginalis is present, trophozoites (the parasite's active form) will be visible in the sample. This is a quick and low-cost option.

• Trichomonas vaginalis can be grown from a swab of vaginal or urethral discharge in a culture media. It could be a few days before the findings of this procedure are accessible.

• NAATs, or nucleic acid amplification tests, are used to identify the parasite's DNA. These tests are highly sensitive and specific, and their use in the diagnosis of trichomoniasis is on the rise.

• Some rapid diagnostic tests can deliver results right at the point of care, which means patients can get an accurate diagnosis and treatment much more quickly thanks to these innovations.

Trichomoniasis symptoms may resemble those of other sexually transmitted infections (STIs), including chlamydia and gonorrhea. Because of the importance of prompt diagnosis and treatment, healthcare providers frequently perform many STI tests at once.

It is critical to get checked out by a doctor if you have been exposed to trichomoniasis or think you might have trichomoniasis. Preventing complications and spreading the virus to other sexual partners, early detection and treatment do more than just ease symptoms. It is also important to educate and treat sexual partners to prevent reinfection.

CHAPTER TWO
Effects And Complications

If neglected, trichomoniasis can have serious consequences, especially for women. Untreated trichomoniasis can cause the following problems and side effects:

•   Individuals with untreated trichomoniasis have a higher risk of contracting additional STIs, including HIV, chlamydia, and gonorrhea. Because trichomoniasis can induce inflammation and irritation, it can pave the way for other diseases to enter the body.

• Trichomoniasis, if left untreated, can cause or exacerbate pelvic inflammatory disease in women. In PID, the uterus, fallopian tubes, and ovaries are all infected, which can have devastating effects on a woman's ability to have children. Chronic pelvic pain is a possible outcome, as can infertility.

• Untreated trichomoniasis in pregnant women has been linked to an increased risk of preterm birth and low birth weight in their infants. Both the mother and the child are at risk from these circumstances.

• When the vaginal environment is altered by trichomoniasis, other infections including bacterial vaginosis (BV) and yeast infections (candidiasis) are more likely to take hold.

• Untreated trichomoniasis patients increase the spread of the parasite because they unwittingly infect their sexual partners.

• Infection that lasts for months or even years without treatment is called chronic trichomoniasis. Repeated episodes of symptoms and consequences are possible outcomes of chronic infections.

• The discomfort and emotional distress caused by trichomoniasis symptoms such vaginal itching, burning, and discharge can drastically reduce a person's quality of life.

If you have trichomoniasis or think you might have it, it's important to consult a doctor very away. Antibiotics such as metronidazole and tinidazole, when administered promptly after a proper diagnosis, are highly efficient at eliminating the parasite and preventing problems. To further assure the virus has been cleared, healthcare practitioners may suggest repeat testing after therapy.

Safe sex practices (frequent, correct condom use), regular STI exams, and communication with sexual partners are all important ways to manage trichomoniasis and lessen its impact on sexual health.

Therapeutics And Administration

Common antibiotics prescribed for trichomoniasis include metronidazole (Flagyl) and tinidazole (Tindamax). The Trichomonas vaginalis parasite can be eliminated and symptoms can be alleviated with the help of these drugs.

Here is the standard protocol for dealing with trichomoniasis:

1. Trichomoniasis is treated with antibiotics prescribed by a doctor.

Antibiotics used most frequently to treat trichomoniasis include:

• The most widely prescribed treatment for trichomoniasis is metronidazole (Flagyl). One high dose or a shorter duration of multiple smaller doses are both possible. While taking metronidazole, as well as for at least 48 hours after finishing your treatment, you should abstain from alcohol.

• The alternative drug tinidazole (Tindamax) is effective against trichomoniasis. Tinidazole, like metronidazole, should not be taken with alcoholic beverages.

2. Involving and informing your sexual partner(s) about your condition and therapy is essential. Trichomoniasis testing and treatment is recommended for both partners to stop reinfection and spread of the parasite.

3. After finishing an antibiotic course of therapy, it is wise to get retested to make sure the infection has been completely eradicated. This is of utmost significance if you suffered from symptoms or a very severe or prolonged infection.

4. You and your partner(s) should refrain from sexual activity until you and your partner(s) have finished treatment for trichomoniasis and tested negative for the illness. This aids in the suppression of reinfection and further spread.

5. When further care is needed, it may be because trichomoniasis has caused problems like pelvic inflammatory disease (PID) or because other STIs are present at the same time.

Your doctor will evaluate the situation and treat any health problems they find.

6. Preventative Measures: Safe sexual behavior is essential for reducing the spread of trichomoniasis and other sexually transmitted infections.

Among these measures are reducing the number of sexual partners and using condoms correctly and consistently when engaging in sexual activity. Key preventative strategies also include routine STI testing and honest discussion of STI status with sexual partners.

7. Sexually active people and those with several sexual partners should get tested for STIs on a regular basis. Complications from trichomoniasis and other STIs can be avoided with prompt diagnosis and treatment.

Keep in mind that trichomoniasis is a curable ailment; those who get the right antibiotics usually get better completely. Even if your symptoms improve before the antibiotic treatment is over, it is still important to finish the full course of medication as directed to eliminate the infection completely.

Get checked out right away if you think you have trichomoniasis or have been exposed to the infection.

CHAPTER THREE
Prevention

Like other sexually transmitted infections (STIs), trichomoniasis can be avoided with preventative measures. The following are some tried-and-true methods for avoiding trichomoniasis:

1. Stay away from sexually risky activities.

• The only foolproof defense against trichomoniasis and other sexually transmitted infections is to refrain from sexual activity.

• Limit the number of sexual partners you have if you are sexually active; doing so reduces your likelihood of contracting sexually transmitted infections.

2. Make regular and proper use of condoms:

• The risk of trichomoniasis and other STIs can be greatly reduced by using condoms, either latex or polyurethane, consistently and correctly during sexual intercourse.

• Remember that condoms may not offer complete protection if they do not fit well, slip, break, or are otherwise misused.

3. Shared monogamy:

• The risk of trichomoniasis and other STIs can be lowered by only engaging in sexual activity within a monogamous relationship where both partners have been tested and found to be STI-free.

4. Routine testing for sexually transmitted infections:

• If you engage in sexual activity, you should think about getting tested for trichomoniasis and other prevalent STIs on a frequent basis, even if you don't feel sick. The key to avoiding problems and spreading the disease is prompt diagnosis and treatment.

• Urge anybody you have sex with to be tested for sexually transmitted diseases.

5. Oral and Anual Sexual Health:

•   Trichomoniasis can be spread through oral and anal sex as well as the more common vaginal and penile routes. Protect yourself from sexually transmitted diseases by always using a condom during oral sex and a dental dam during anal intercourse.

6. Don't become horny while drunk or high:

• Risky sexual activities, such as unprotected sex, can result from the impaired judgment brought on by alcohol and drugs. Substance use should be avoided during sexual relations to lower the risk of sexually transmitted infections.

7. Talking & Telling the Truth:

• It's important for people to talk openly and honestly with their sexual partners about their STI status, their testing history, and safer sex practices. Prompt partners to come clean about any diseases they may have and be open about your own.

8. Hygiene of Oneself:

• Genital infections can be avoided by practicing good personal hygiene, which includes regular genital cleansing. Cleanliness is certainly important, but it's not enough to make sexual activity risk-free.

9. Knowledge and understanding:

• Seek reputable information from healthcare practitioners, educational resources, and public health organizations to learn more about trichomoniasis and other sexually transmitted infections. Understanding the dangers and how to avoid them gives you more control over your life.

In other people, the trichomoniasis infection may not even cause any obvious symptoms. Therefore, it is crucial to take precautions even if neither you nor your spouse is currently experiencing symptoms.

You should get tested for trichomoniasis and get treatment if you have it, and you should tell your sexual partner(s) if you think they may have been exposed to the infection.

The Reality Of Trichomoniasis

Having to deal with the discomfort of trichomoniasis symptoms can make daily life difficult. Fortunately, trichomoniasis is a medically manageable infection, and most patients make good recoveries after receiving treatment. Some important considerations for those dealing with trichomoniasis are as follows:

• Seek Medical Help If you have been diagnosed with trichomoniasis or think you might have the condition, it is crucial that you get treatment right away. Antibiotic treatment is usually necessary to eradicate the parasite and alleviate the symptoms of trichomoniasis.

• Take all of the antibiotics your doctor prescribes, whether it's metronidazole or tinidazole, and finish the full course. Even if your symptoms improve before the antibiotic treatment is over, it is vital that you finish the whole course of medication. That way, the disease is more likely to be wiped out completely.

• It is crucial to refrain from sexual activity while being treated for trichomoniasis, since this will help to avoid the spread of the infection to other sexual partners. Share this information with your sexual partners so they can get checked out and treated if necessary.

• After finishing treatment, it's a good idea to get checked again to make sure the infection is completely gone.

This is especially crucial if your infection was serious or persisted for an extended period of time and you experienced symptoms.

• Practice safe sex by always and properly using condoms to avoid re-infection and the spread of sexually transmitted diseases. Reducing the number of sexual partners is important, as is considering mutual monogamy with people who have both passed STI tests.

• Keeping up with frequent genital cleansing is an important part of practicing proper personal hygiene and preventing genital infections. Cleanliness is certainly important, but it's not enough to make sexual activity risk-free.

• Inform yourself about trichomoniasis and other sexually transmitted diseases. You may better protect your sexual health by making educated decisions when it comes to condom use, STI prevention practices, and the frequency with which you get tested.

• Complications from trichomoniasis, such as pelvic inflammatory disease (PID) and other concomitant STIs, should be addressed as soon as possible by working with your healthcare professional and following their recommended treatment programs.

• Emotional support: Dealing with a sexually transmitted infection (STI) like trichomoniasis can be difficult. If you feel like you need to talk to someone, seek out those who can offer you assistance, such as friends, family, or healthcare experts. People with STIs can find comfort in the fact that there are local and online support groups for them to join.

Know that you are not alone in coping with trichomoniasis because it is a prevalent STI. You can effectively manage and finally overcome trichomoniasis by combining medical treatment with responsible sexual conduct and open conversation with sexual partners.

Conclusion

Finally, Trichomonas vaginalis is responsible for the widespread STI known as trichomoniasis. Symptoms include vaginal discharge, itching, burning, and discomfort during sex because it primarily affects the genital and urinary tracts. However, many people who have trichomoniasis may not experience any symptoms at all.

Laboratory testing, including microscopic examination, culture, and nucleic acid amplification tests, are used to diagnose trichomoniasis. The infection can be cured and further difficulties avoided if medicines like metronidazole or tinidazole are administered promptly and as prescribed.

Seeking medical attention, finishing the complete course of medications, and engaging in safe sex are all important responsibilities for those living with trichomoniasis. Managing a sexually transmitted illness requires being honest with sexual partners, learning as much as can about STIs, and treating any difficulties that may arise.

Trichomoniasis is curable, and people can recover from it without compromising their sexual health if they take the correct steps. The public health burden of trichomoniasis and other STIs can be minimized by prevention, early identification, and responsible sexual conduct.

THE END